FROM FACTORY TO TABLE
WHAT YOU'RE REALLY EATING™

THE TRUTH BEHIND ANTIBIOTICS, PESTICIDES, AND HORMONES

KATHARINA SMUNDAK

rosen publishing's
rosen
central®

New York

Published in 2018 by The Rosen Publishing Group, Inc.
29 East 21st Street, New York, NY 10010

First Edition

Library of Congress Cataloging-in-Publication Data

Names: Smundak, Katharina, author.
Title: The truth behind antibiotics, pesticides, and hormones / Katharina Smundak.
Description: New York : Rosen Central, 2018. | Series: From factory to table: what you're really eating | Audience: Grades 5–8. | Includes bibliographical references and index.
Identifiers: LCCN 2017019020| ISBN 9781499439229 (library bound) | ISBN 9781499439199 (pbk.) | ISBN 9781499439212 (6 pack)
Subjects: LCSH: Antibiotics—Juvenile literature. | Antibiotics in agriculture—Juvenile literature. | Pesticides—Juvenile literature. | Hormones—Juvenile literature.
Classification: LCC RM267 .S59 2018 | DDC 615.3/29—dc23
LC record available at https://lccn.loc.gov/2017019020

Manufactured in China

CONTENTS

In the last couple of generations, the average person has moved away from the farm. Most of us get our food from the supermarket, and so it is easy to forget to think about where our food comes from and how it ends up in our home. Although food is fundamental for human survival, we know little about the complex process involved in its production and the decisions that farmers and governments make to grow the food we eat. In short, we are fairly disconnected from food production. But in the last couple of years, people have become increasingly concerned about food: how it is produced, what substances are involved in its production, and what effects these substances have on our bodies and on our environment. Basically, we are learning that when we eat an orange, we are not just eating an orange, and when we eat steak, that is not the only thing we are ingesting. These are important questions to ask. After all, we are what we eat.

Antibiotics, pesticides, and hormones play important roles in growing the food that we eat. In one way or another, they help farmers produce greater quantities of food than they would be able to produce without them. And yet, we see more and more labels on our food indicating that it is hormone free or that the animals were not treated with antibiotics. These labels are introduced because these substances can negatively affect our health.

In order to understand the labels on our food, people must understand exactly what antibiotics, pesticides, and hormones are. They must also understand what role they play in our food supply, how we come into contact with them, and the consequences

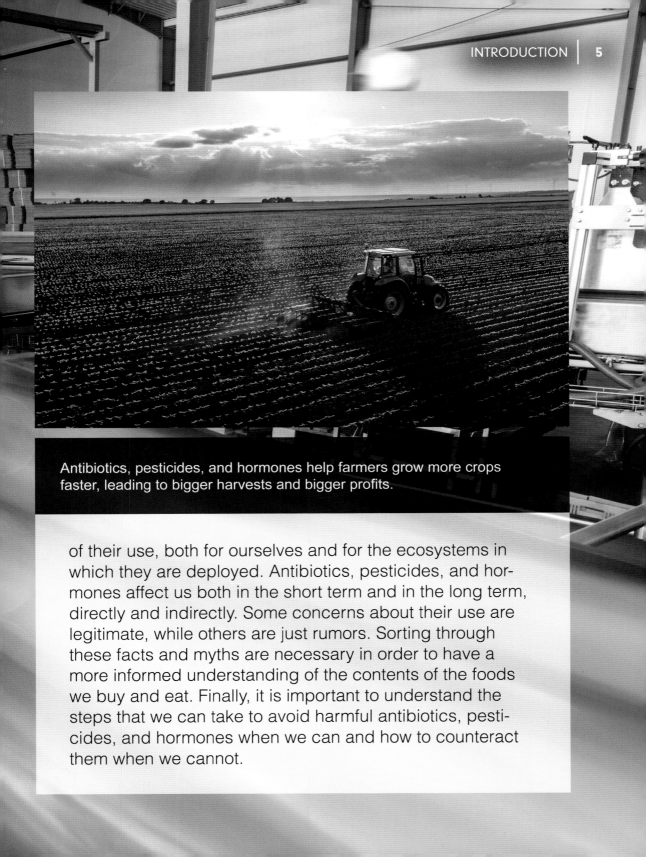

Antibiotics, pesticides, and hormones help farmers grow more crops faster, leading to bigger harvests and bigger profits.

of their use, both for ourselves and for the ecosystems in which they are deployed. Antibiotics, pesticides, and hormones affect us both in the short term and in the long term, directly and indirectly. Some concerns about their use are legitimate, while others are just rumors. Sorting through these facts and myths are necessary in order to have a more informed understanding of the contents of the foods we buy and eat. Finally, it is important to understand the steps that we can take to avoid harmful antibiotics, pesticides, and hormones when we can and how to counteract them when we cannot.

CHAPTER ONE

ANTIBIOTICS, PESTICIDES, AND HORMONES, OH MY!

O ur planet's population is already high, and it is rising. Since we all need food to live, farmers are faced with the task of growing the food we need to survive. Since the 1960s in particular, when Earth's population started booming and famine for millions of people became a real threat, farmers, governments, and scientists have worked together to find ways to grow a maximal amount of food given limited resources. Three important tools have been used in agriculture in the twentieth century to achieve maximal outputs, such as bigger crop yields or heavier animals, while using minimal inputs, such as less feed for animals, for example. These tools are antibiotics, pesticides, and hormones. While these tools do perform these functions, there are significant risks associated with them for humans, for animals, and for the greater environment. To understand the potential risks these tools may pose to humans and our environment, we must know exactly what antibiotics, hormones, and pesticides are and why they can be problematic.

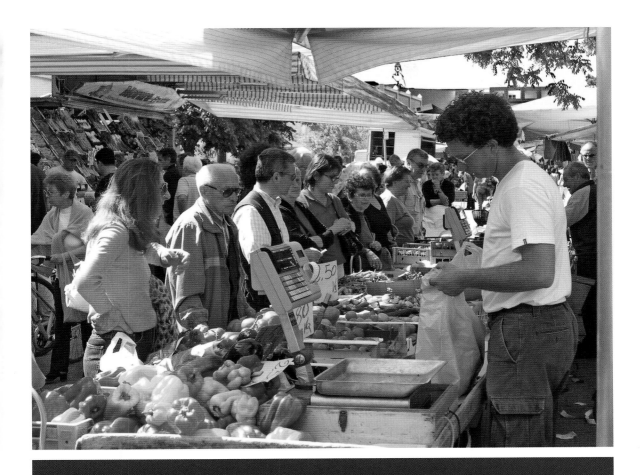

With so many people in the world, farmers and governments have to figure out ways to feed everyone.

ANTIBIOTICS: MY, HOW YOU'VE GROWN!

Most people are familiar with antibiotics as the medication they take when they are sick with a stomach bug or a sore throat. The discovery of antibiotics in the twentieth century has saved millions

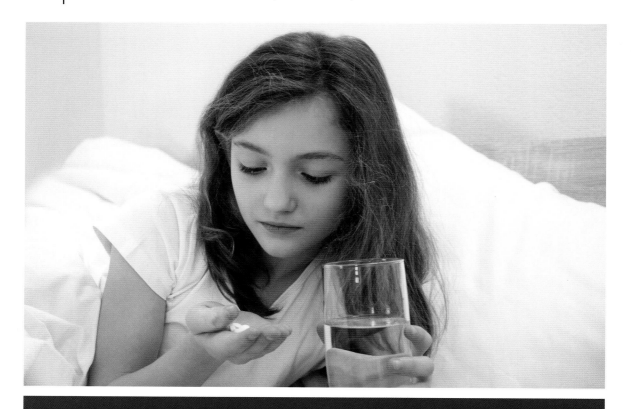

Antibiotics probably bring to mind being sick. Doctors prescribe antibiotics to people to help them battle illnesses.

and millions of lives. Antibiotics kill bacteria. Antibiotics are produced from bacteria, molds, and fungi.

In September 1928, Sir Alexander Fleming, a professor of bacteriology at St. Mary's Hospital in London, went on vacation. When he came back, he inspected the petri dishes on which he had started growing the Staphylococcus bacteria before his vacation. Bacterial colonies dotted his petri dishes, but he noticed something strange about one of them: a mold had contaminated it and no colonies grew directly around it. This mold, it later turned out, was penicillin, and it prevented bacteria from growing.

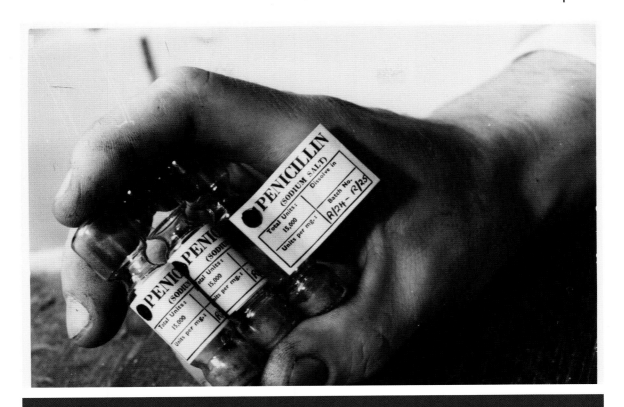

Penicillin is one of the most famous and widely used antibiotics. It has saved millions and millions of lives.

From there, a scientist named Howard Florey and others working at Oxford University started developing methods to make penicillin available on a large scale. It was first used to treat a bacterial infection in 1940 and saved many lives during World War II. Infection had always been a bigger killer during war than injuries. As Howard Markel writes in the 2013 article "The Real Story behind Penicillin," during World War I alone, 18 percent of soldiers had died of bacterial pneumonia. Thanks to penicillin, during World War II, that number fell to a mere 1 percent!

Just like humans, animals can also get bacterial infections. This is one reason farmers give them antibiotics. But another reason for antibiotics in agriculture is to promote growth. Farmers use growth-promoting antibiotics (GPAs) to make animals gain weight faster and enhance growth and feed efficiency. Then, animals require less food to gain weight. GPAs are given to animals in low doses, which means the dose is not high enough to kill all the bacteria. As a result, bacteria not killed by the small dose of antibiotics reproduce and pass on their resistance to future generations and crowd out bacteria that are killed by antibiotics. According to the Centers for Disease Control and Prevention (CDC), these antibiotic-resistant bacteria can enter our food supply as the bacteria can contaminate the meat of the slaughtered animals. Animal waste containing these resistant bacteria can be found in fertilizer or in water that is later used on crops. These bacteria then can remain on the crops that humans eat at home. If people become infected with antibiotic-resistant bacteria, doctors may need to prescribe stronger antibiotics to kill the bacteria. At some point, bacteria may develop resistance to all known antibiotics, and humans may no longer have antibiotics strong enough to fight the bacteria. Antibiotic-resistant bacteria can be deadly.

PESTICIDES: A MIXED BAG

Pesticides can also be harmful to humans. Pesticides are substances that prevent, repel, or destroy pests, which can come in the form of insects, weeds, fungi, and rodents. Correspondingly, pesticides can be insecticides, herbicides, fungicides, or rodenticides. They are used in gardens and in homes, but they are also applied on a massive scale to crops. As of 2004, over one billion pounds of pesticides were used in the United States alone. In industrial agriculture, they are sprayed on crops as a kind of mist.

Pesticides enter the food chain in multiple ways. The first way is direct: they are applied to the crops that humans eat. Because they are sprayed, wind can also carry pesticides through the air into rivers or other farms. Furthermore, they can enter our water by seeping through the soil and entering groundwater. They can also remain on the surface of the ground and enter our water supply as part of surface runoff, which is the flow of water over land. Runoff is basically when excessive water travels over land to a river, because of either too much rain or melting snow.

For humans, pesticides are dangerous because they can act as endocrine disruptors (EDs), which are chemicals our bodies respond to like hormones. They are very likely to be carcinogenic, or cancer causing, in humans. According to the Environmental Protection Agency (EPA), EDs not only increase the risk of cancer, they also interfere with reproduction, disturb nervous and immune system function, and affect development. In an article titled "Health Effects of Chronic Pesticide Exposure," researchers Michael C. R. Alavanja, Jane A. Hoppin, and Freya Kamel present evidence that people who are consistently exposed to pesticides, such as people who spray crops, have higher rates of certain cancers as well as problems with their nervous systems, livers, and motor function (which is their ability to control how their body moves). Exposure to pesticides has also been linked to Parkinson's disease, although this problem seems to affect primarily people who work directly with pesticides, such as farmers. Some endocrine-disrupting pesticides have also been linked to type 2 diabetes. Again though, like with hormones, it's not clear whether the endocrine disruptor levels found in the wild are high enough to affect humans. Scientists are considering the environment as a factor because cancer rates, for example, are rising.

HORMONES: NOT JUST FOR TEENAGERS

Hormones are another substance sometimes given to animals to promote growth. They are chemical messengers that regulate various biochemical reactions. In humans, they play an important role in reproduction, growth, and energy regulation. In the United States, steroids are given to cattle and sheep in order to make them grow faster and transform the food they're eating into fat and muscle more efficiently. Steroids in pellet form are attached surgically to the back of cattle ears. This implant slowly dissolves over the course of the animal's life as the steroids enter its blood stream. These ears are then discarded once the animal is slaughtered. In the United States, hormones are not approved for use in chickens, as it is difficult to give hormones to a chicken on a routine. So when chicken is "hormone-free" at the supermarket, it's true (but technically it's true for all chickens!). A growth hormone called recombinant bovine growth hormone (rBGH) is also given to dairy cows to increase their milk production. Like antibiotic-resistant bacteria, hormones can end up in our bodies indirectly both through the food we eat or through animal waste, which often enters our water supply.

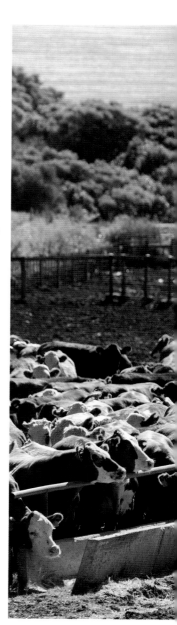

In the United States, cattle used for meat are treated with six hormones, three of which are natural and three of which are synthetic (meaning they are manufactured in a lab, not produced naturally). All six of them are banned in the European Union (EU). Indeed, hormone-treated beef is illegal in the EU and has not been allowed for import since 1999. That year, the EU's Scientific Committee on Veterinary Measures Relating to Public Health

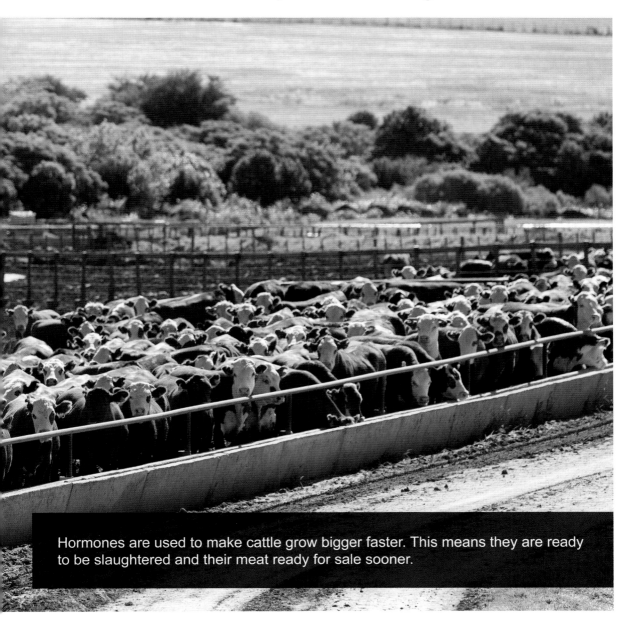

Hormones are used to make cattle grow bigger faster. This means they are ready to be slaughtered and their meat ready for sale sooner.

published a report that concluded that hormones had potentially negative hormonal and developmental effects, among others.

Like pesticides, synthetic hormones are endocrine disruptors. The milk of cows treated with a hormone called rBGH contains higher levels of another hormone called IGF-1, which has been found to fuel tumor growth. That said, IGF-1 has also been found in people who drink soy milk, which is not produced by cows at all. As a result, the American Cancer Society has no official position on rBGH. In the end, the danger of hormones depends on the quantities in which they're consumed. In a child that hasn't yet gone through puberty, these small quantities of hormones could have stronger effects than on an adult. The hormone levels in the meat we eat are a fraction of the hormone levels we produce ourselves, so whether or not hormone-treated meat is bad for humans is a subject of debate.

MYTH

Hormone-free beef is healthier and more natural.

FACT

All cattle produce hormones naturally! Although, for example, cattle treated with hormones have more estrogen than those not implanted with steroid pellets, the quantity of estrogen per serving that we end up eating is less than is found in the same serving of eggs and miniscule relative to the amount of estrogen our bodies produce.

MYTH

Organic farms do not use pesticides.

FACT

All farms use pesticides. The difference is that organic farmers use pesticides that are derived from natural products and not created in a lab. The fact that it comes from a natural source does not mean that it is not harmful for us or for the environment.

MYTH

There are traces of antibiotics in animals treated with antibiotics.

FACT

Before meat can be sold on the market, all antibiotic residue must be gone from the animal, which means that there is a withdrawal period prior to slaughter during which the animals are not given any food containing antibiotics.

CHAPTER TWO

DIRECT EFFECTS ON HUMANS

Although their use is common in producing the food that humans eat, few people truly understand the effects of antibiotics, pesticides, or hormones on the human body. Understanding how these things affect our bodies is an important part of making informed decisions about what food products to buy. Let's start with antibiotics.

We've established that the biggest problem with the consistent use of antibiotic in animals is that it creates antibiotic-resistant bacteria. But where does antibiotic resistance come from? The point of antibiotics is to kill bacteria in some way or another. They work by attacking those parts of bacterial cells that differ from human cells. Human cells, for example, don't have cell walls, while bacterial cells do, so some antibiotics prevent bacteria from building walls. Bacterial cells also have different cell membrane structures, copy their DNA differently, and build proteins differently. To fight bacteria, some antibiotics dissolve only bacterial cell membranes, while others attack how the bacteria copy their DNA or build their proteins.

However, imagine that in this group of bacteria that is hit by antibiotics, there are a couple that cannot be killed by this

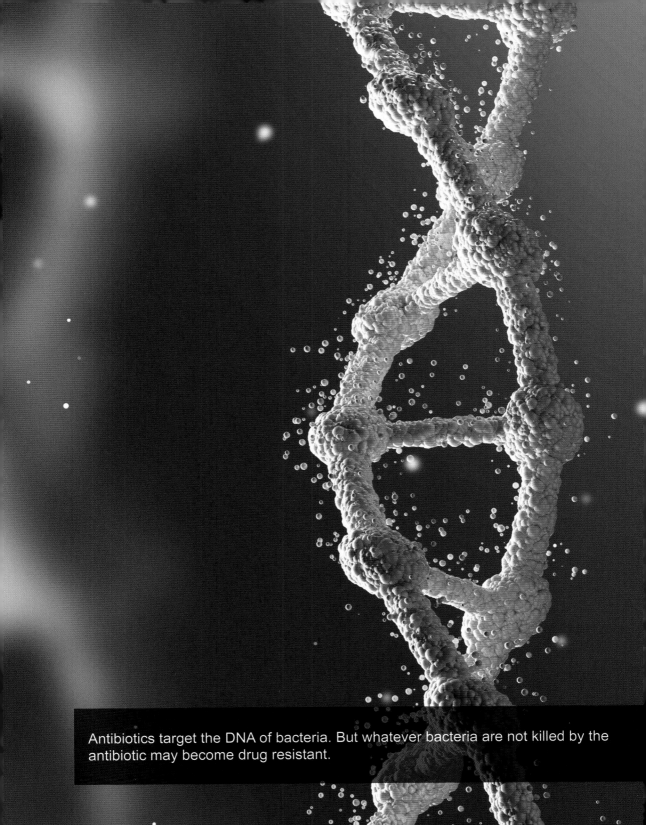

Antibiotics target the DNA of bacteria. But whatever bacteria are not killed by the antibiotic may become drug resistant.

antibiotic because of some mutation in their DNA. They survive while all the other bacteria die. They reproduce, and so they pass on their resistant genes to the next generation. As a result, the next generation of bacteria will require a stronger antibiotic to kill it.

THE BIG THREE BACTERIA

The infection-causing bacteria in food that present the greatest threat to humans are *Escherichia coli* (most commonly known as *E. coli*), *Salmonella*, and *Campylobacter*. Some *E. coli* strains are present in our lower intestines, and they cause us no harm at all. Other strains, however, are the causes of foodborne illnesses. Normally, eating food contaminated with *E. coli* causes food poisoning, but it can also have more serious consequences. It can be avoided by cooking meat so it is not raw and washing produce properly. In 2011, a particular strain of *E. coli* in Germany led to the deaths of several people and hospitalized hundreds of others. Eating food contaminated by this strain of *E. coli*, O104:H4, caused bloody diarrhea and in some cases led to deadly kidney failure. According to an August 2011 *Scientific American* article "*E. coli* on the March," this particular strain was resistant to at least fourteen antibiotics! This resistance had to develop in the presence of many antibiotics, like at a hospital or on a farm.

Salmonella is another bacterium that can cause food poisoning. Like with *E. coli*, humans can be infected with *Salmonella* by eating improperly cooked meat that is still a little raw. It can also be found in raw eggs, raw milk, and on produce washed with water that contains the bacteria. The symptoms of *Salmonella* poisoning are fever, stomach cramps, and diarrhea, which can lead to dehydration. For healthy adults, *Salmonella* poisoning is not life-threatening. However, it is dangerous and even fatal for old people, children, and babies. In addition, if the infection spreads from the intestines to the blood stream, it becomes typhoid fever. While *Salmonella* poisoning generally doesn't require antibiotics for treatment, typhoid does. That's where antibiotic resistance becomes an issue.

The danger of *Campylobacter* is the same as that of *Salmonella*: eating food contaminated with it leads to campylobacteriosis. The symptoms are similar to *Salmonella* poisoning: diarrhea, fever, and stomach cramps. Campylobacteriosis comes from eating undercooked contaminated chicken. Other meats,

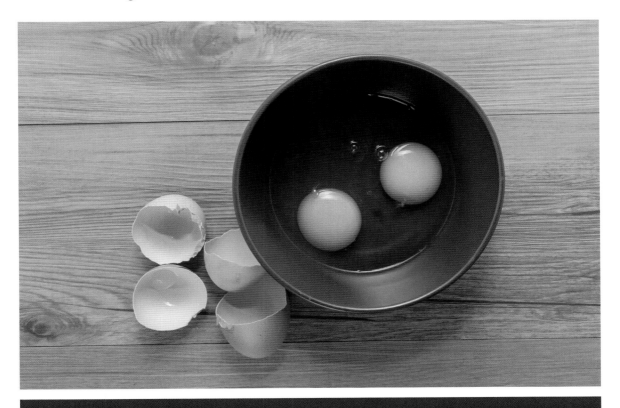

Raw eggs can have *E. coli*. It is important always to cook eggs and not eat them raw. This is the best way to avoid getting sick.

such as pork or contaminated milk and water, can also cause an infection. Most of the time, no treatment is required, but for people with weak immune systems—such as children, the elderly, or those with an immunodeficiency—the infection can be very serious and require antibiotic treatment. The use of antibiotics in the animals we eat has led to the evolution of antibiotic-resistant *Campylobacter.*

DISRUPTING AND CORRUPTING

When it comes to some synthetic hormones and pesticides, they disrupt the endocrine system in various ways. The endocrine system is the collection of glands that secrete hormones: the pituitary and the pineal glands in the brain; the thyroid gland in the neck; the adrenal gland above the kidneys; the pancreas, located behind the stomach; and the ovaries in women and the testes in men. The endocrine system refers to these glands as well as to the hormones themselves.

According to the EPA, the body responds to endocrine disruptors in different ways. The body responds to some endocrine disruptors as it would to a hormone since it can't tell the difference between the two. There are two possible outcomes. One is an over-response. For example, if the body receives a growth hormone, it will lead to more muscle mass. The other outcome is a response at the wrong time, such as producing insulin when it's not needed. Other endocrine disruptors block hormone receptors. Finally, others "directly stimulate or inhibit the endocrine system and cause overproduction or underproduction of hormones," which means that they either push the endocrine system to respond or prevent the endocrine system from responding and thus cause it to produce either too many or too few hormones.

DIETHYLSTILBESTROL (DES)

In the 1930s, scientists developed diethylstilbestrol (DES), a synthetic estrogen. From 1940 to 1971, it was prescribed to pregnant women to prevent miscarriages, or the usually unwanted loss of pregnancy. In that time period, it was, according to the CDC, prescribed to somewhere between five and ten million women. By the late 1960s, doctors noticed that women whose mothers had taken DES while pregnant with them were likelier to have a certain kind of cancer. Indeed, DES caused this cancer. These women were also likelier to miscarry and to deliver premature babies. In 1971, the Food and Drug Administration (FDA) banned DES. It is now considered an endocrine disruptor.

Endocrine disruptors can play a particularly important and negative role during important and sensitive stages in the life cycle like pregnancy, development, and lactation. Endocrine disruptors are also considered a reason for widespread cases of puberty, a time of intense hormonal activity during a child's development, starting earlier than normal. In the past, for example, girls on average started developing breasts around age eleven. In a May 2015 article in *Scientific American* titled "Early Puberty: Cause and Effects," Dina Fine Maron reports many cases of girls as young as seven developing breasts. Although obesity is considered the leading cause of this phenomenon, scientists now think that endocrine disruptors, among them some pesticides, also play a part. These endocrine disruptors mimic estrogen. They bind with estrogen-receptors, which control the expression of certain genes, in cells. Estrogen plays an important role in puberty, so when an endocrine disruptor that mimics estrogen is present in the body, it can trigger breast growth or an early menstrual period, which is linked to breast cancer.

The case of polybrominated biphenyl (PBB) in 1973 in Michigan is another good example of the negative effects of EDs on humans. At the time, PBB, a flame retardant and an estrogen-mimicking chemical, was accidentally added to cattle

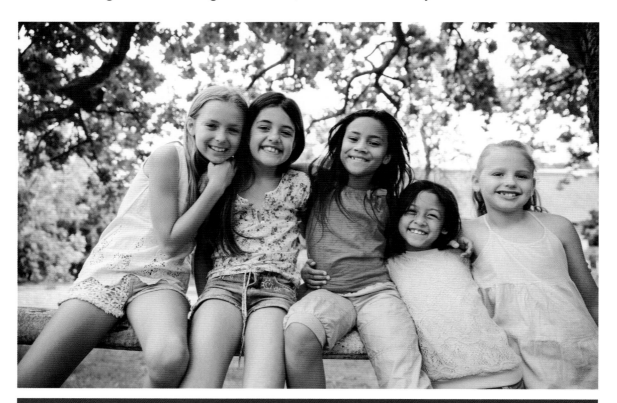

Everybody is different and girls hit puberty at different times. However, there has been a larger trend of girls hitting puberty earlier.

feed. The daughters of the pregnant women who ate the beef that came from these cattle and drank their milk started their periods significantly earlier than normal. PBB is not a pesticide or a synthetic hormone, but it is a good example of the effects of EDs on the endocrine system and, by extension, on development. In addition to pesticides, a common ingredient in hard plastics called bisphenol A (BPA) is also an ED. Again, though, EDs are not the only factor in early puberty.

Although some people are concerned that early exposure to estrogen could increase the risk of cancer in women, perhaps the bigger issue with early puberty is its social effect on young girls. In a March 2012 article in the *New York Times* titled "Puberty Before Age 10: A New Normal?" Elizabeth Weil writes about the consequences of early puberty for girls. Girls who develop earlier than their peers are likelier to have lower self-esteem and eating disorders. Early development is also linked to depression and higher-risk sexual activity. Girls who look older than they are often are treated as if they were older than they are, and, therefore, they face increased social pressure.

We have seen the negative ways that antibiotic-resistant bacteria, antibiotic use in animals, and endocrine-disrupting hormones and pesticides affect the human body. These three factors also have indirect impacts on humans through their effects on our environment.

CHAPTER THREE

THE BIGGER PICTURE

Pesticides, antibiotic-resistant bacteria, and hormones can reach us directly, either through the food we eat that has been treated with them or through the water we drink that has been polluted by them. But those are not the only ways that they can affect us. Pesticides and hormones in particular have an impact on the environment—which is another way they indirectly affect us.

PESTICIDES AND HORMONES ARE HERE TO STAY

Bioaccumulation is one of the reasons that pesticides and synthetic hormones pose a threat. Bioaccumulation is the accumulation of a substance in an organism. It occurs when more of a substance remains in the body than the body gets rid of, either through excretion or by breaking the substance down. As a result, the substance builds up in the organism. Substances that are persistent, bioaccumulative, and toxic are known as PBTs or persistent organic pollutants (POPs). Pesticides are a good example of them. POPs are

24

particularly dangerous because they move up the food chain. When a creature low on the food chain, such as a clam, consumes a POP, it does not stay just in that clam. If a fish eats that clam, the POP will become concentrated in the fish. The higher up an animal is on the food chain, the greater the concentration of the POP in that animal. This is called biomagnification.

Because humans are at the top of our food chain, we end up eating high concentrations of POPs. The case of DDT is a good example. DDT (dichloro-diphenyl-trychloroethane) was the first modern pesticide, developed in the 1940s. It was and continues to be used to fight typhus and malaria. In the past, it was also used as an agricultural insecticide. However, increased insect resistance to DDT as well as the publication of Rachel Carson's book *Silent Spring*, which drew attention to the negative effects of DDT on the environment and bird populations, caused it to be banned as an insecticide in 1972.

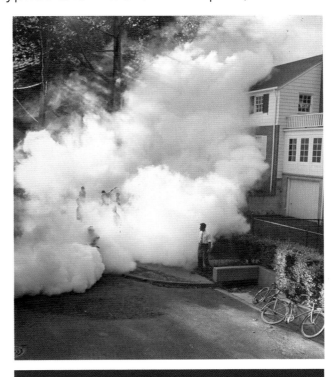

Despite the fact that DDT has been banned for more than thirty years, it is still a threat because it is a POP. Certain types of fish caught in Washington, for example, still contain DDT. Pregnant women and breastfeeding women are warned against eating such fish, as DDT

When DDT was first introduced, everyone thought it was safe. It would even be sprayed on people!

can be passed from mother to child through breast milk. DDT exposure can cause cognitive problems, and the EPA lists it as a possible carcinogen (like other pesticides previously discussed). The FDA warns that fish grown on fish farms are also vulnerable to pesticide bioaccumulation since the food they eat may have these substances stored in their fatty tissues, where POPs are generally stored.

Scientists started considering the dangers of DDT and other pesticides for humans once they noticed their negative effect on birds. Animals' negative reactions to substances introduced into the environment by humans can be a warning that these substances are also dangerous for us, too. Humans must not ignore other creatures' responses to the substances we introduce into the ecosystem. As such, we should pay attention to the hormones that we introduce into our water supply, including those that come from the manure of cattle treated with steroids. These hormones have clear effects on fish. In a 2015 article published in *Nature Communications*, a team of researchers concluded that hormones that enter water supplies from cattle farms had lowered reproductive rates in fish and altered their endocrine system, among other effects. Not only does this mean a smaller fish population—and thus, a smaller food supply for other animals and humans—but it also warns humans about the impact of these hormones if consumed.

WHERE WOULD WE BEE WITHOUT YOU?

The use of pesticides is also linked to declines in bee, butterfly, and earthworm populations. Although we generally do not eat these animals, bees and earthworms in particular play very important parts in our food supply. Bees are pollinators; they are the means by which certain plants reproduce. Bees take pollen from the male part of a plant and apply it to the female part of another plant. That plant can then produce a seed. This seed becomes the next generation of the plant. Crops from alfalfa to cotton to tomatoes and cucumbers to almonds rely on pollination to reproduce. According to the UN Food and Agriculture Organization, bees pollinate seventy-one of the one hundred crops that provide 90 percent of human's food!

As bee populations decline, scientists are looking into what may be causing this very serious problem. In the European Union, the use of a certain class of insecticides known as neonicotinoids has been banned because of a suspected link between this pesticide and bee colony decline. So far, the

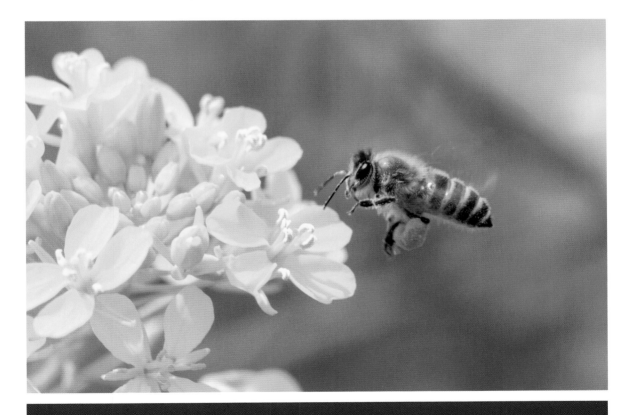

Bees are incredibly important to food production. It is important to protect them and pesticides are a big threat.

evidence for this relationship is not conclusive. Some studies have concluded that neonicotinoids do negatively affect bees. Others have argued that such studies exposed bees to higher levels of the pesticide than they would encounter in nature. Moreover, other factors contribute to bee decline, including parasites, disease, poor nutrition, and climate change.

Regardless of what research says about neonicotinoids, the EU's ban has led to the use of other pesticides instead. Neonicotinoids are popular because they are much less harmful than previous generations of pesticides, including organophosphates, which are much more toxic to both humans and animals. A study by the Royal Holloway University of London showed that another class of pesticides known as pyrethroids reduced bees' size, which made them worse at collecting pollen and nectar. Insecticides are designed to kill insects, so it is no surprise that they have an effect on bees. The questions scientists must ask are,

SHOULD YOU BELIEVE THE BUZZ?

Growing awareness and concern about agricultural practices has led people to come to conclusions that are not always supported by evidence. Neonicotinoids, for example, were cited in many mainstream newspapers as the only reason for bee death, when, in fact, there are many factors that play a role in bee colony decline, especially when you take into consideration how complex ecosystems are. It is usually very difficult to isolate one factor as a cause of a problem when there are many factors at play.

"How much insecticide can we safely use?" and, "What insecticides do the least harm to bees while still being effective for pests?"

It is, of course, important to pay attention to what we introduce into the environment. We are all part of one ecosystem. But rather than panic or make hasty diet changes, a smart eater will do their own research. Everybody is guilty of spreading information about subjects they haven't fully researched, because they've heard friends talking about it or saw something about it on TV. That knowledge can be a good starting point, but it's important to check reliable resources and know the facts.

EARTHWORMS: NATURE'S FARMHAND

Pesticides also affect earthworms. Earthworms play a really important part in soil health. Soil health is, of course, important for plant growth and productivity. Earthworms eat dead organisms and plant matter. They then excrete it as cast, which contains nitrogen and phosphate—key nutrients to help plants grow. Basically, earthworms create fertilizer for plants. Earthworms also build air pockets in soil, which make it easier for water to reach a plant's roots and create space for roots to grow more easily. A soil ecosystem can survive without earthworms, but their contributions are valuable and help plants grow. (Worms are also an important part of the food chain, meaning that, like fish, their exposure to pesticides affects the animals that eat them, too.)

Pesticide use harms earthworms by lowering their reproduction rates and decreasing their size. A 2014 University of Denmark study showed that there were often two to three times more earthworms in soil samples not sprayed with pesticides than in those sprayed with pesticides. Another study concluded that

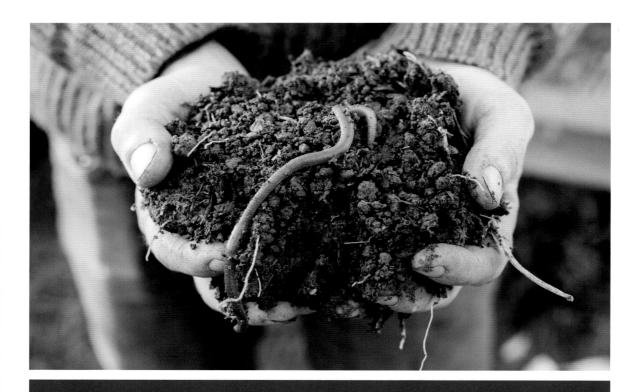

Pesticides are deadly to many living things, including earthworms. These worms play an important role in farming.

some pesticides are toxic to earthworms, even at less than their recommended application doses.

Pesticides play a huge role in agriculture. They kill organisms—such as mites, insects, and weeds—that are hurting the plants farmers want to grow. By doing so, they allow bigger crop yields for human consumption. Farmers often must weigh the benefits and disadvantages of the techniques they use. Pesticide use is a good example of the balance that farmers must strike. Does the benefit of killing the pest and increasing crop yield outweigh the damage done to the ecosystem and risks for humans who consume these foods?

CHAPTER FOUR

STAYING SAFE AND SMART

I t's clear that although antibiotics, pesticides, and hormones play important roles in increasing our food supply, their use can have harmful consequences for our bodies and our planet. However, there are ways to avoid pesticides and hormones as well as the antibiotic-resistant bacteria that use of antibiotics breeds.

WHEN IT COMES TO DIET, KEEP IT SIMPLE

Given that pesticides as well as synthetic hormones act as endocrine disruptors, which have been linked to cancer and reproductive and developmental problems, it is smart to avoid them as much as possible. Make sure to wash and scrub your fruits and vegetables well before eating them, as pesticide residue may remain on them or may have landed on them from another field. After washing them, they should be dried with a cloth. Peeling, when possible, is also a good way to lower the risks of consuming pesticides, as is removing the outer leaves of a leafy vegetable, such as lettuce. The Environmental Working Group's "Shopper's Guide to Pesticides in Produce," published since 2004, lists the fruits and vegetables that, when tested, had the most pesticides on them after preparation (meaning, after having been washed and peeled, where necessary). Strawberries top that list. They are followed by spinach, nectarines, apples, peaches, pears, cherries, grapes, celery, tomatoes, sweet bell peppers, and potatoes. This list does not mean you should not eat fruits and vegetables. It is definitely better to eat fruits and veggies than processed foods, such as chips and cookies. One solution is to eat fruits and vegetables that tested with little to no pesticide residue. The EWG

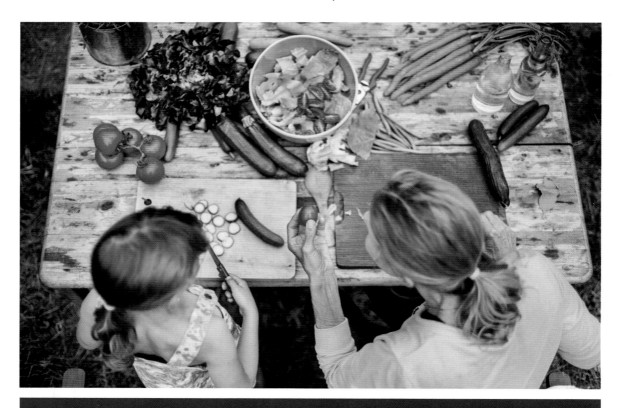

Peeling and washing fruits and vegetables helps get rid of any residue left by pesticides. This should be done even to organic fruits and vegetables.

suggests sweet corn, avocado, pineapples, onions, mango, melon, grapefruit, and cauliflower, among others. The EWG report reflects pesticide loads in conventionally grown produce, not organic.

When it comes to meat, pesticides are often stored in the fat of the meat. Removing the fat before cooking can lower the amount of pesticides present. Also think about where the meat is from. If a cut of salmon comes from the Puget Sound, don't buy it, as there are high DDT levels in fish from that water source. If consumers want to make sure the fish they buy and eat is both healthy and ocean friendly, they can use the Monterey Bay Aquarium's Seafood Watch guide. This free online resource ranks seafood's safety and sustainability based on type, location, and how it was raised. Sure enough, the guide recommends avoiding the Puget Sound's Chinook salmon.

MYTHS ABOUT ORGANIC FOODS

It is very important not to confuse organic with pesticide-free. Organic farmers use pesticides. However, these pesticides are derived from natural sources. They are often less effective than synthetic pesticides and so require higher dosages. A study comparing the use of natural pesticides to synthetic pesticides concluded that the use of natural pesticides required six to seven sprays to get a 75 percent yield, whereas synthetic pesticides required four sprays to get a 90 percent yield.

There is also a common assumption that because pesticides used in organic foods come from natural sources, they are safe and not harmful. That is not true. Two of the most common natural pesticides, copper sulfate and rotenone, degrade slowly. A September 2012 *Scientific American* article titled "Are lower pesticide residues a good reason to buy organic? Probably not" concluded that the copper used in organic farming is less safe for humans than synthetic alternatives. It is also very toxic for birds and earthworms. In "Pesticide/Environmental Exposures and Parkinson's Disease in East Texas," published in the *Journal of Agromedicine*, researchers found that exposure to rotenone increased the risk of Parkinson's disease five-fold when compared to the synthetic alternative, chlorpyrifos.

Although people often think that there are fewer pesticides in organic food, this is simply because many studies only test for synthetic pesticides. They do not always test for the presence of organic pesticides. Ultimately, organic or not, pesticides are pesticides. As a consumer, it is very important not to confuse "organic"

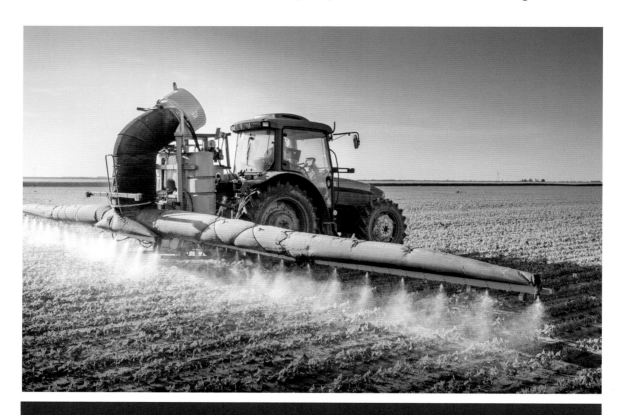

Organic farms use pesticides, too. However, they are natural pesticides. This doesn't mean you shouldn't wash your produce, though.

or "natural" with "healthy," necessarily. One does not guarantee the other. Remember, arsenic is natural, but it is still a poison.

In the case of antibiotic resistance, the CDC provides helpful guidelines. Bacteria are killed when cooked at high temperatures. The government's food safety site indicates the appropriate temperatures that various meats should be cooked to. Poultry should be cooked to 165 degrees Fahrenheit (73 degrees Celsius); ground beef, veal, pork,

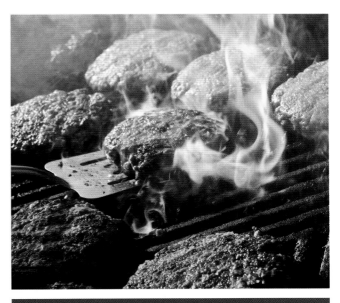

Use a meat thermometer to make sure meat is cooked to the right temperature.

and lamb to 145°F (62°C); and fresh pork and whole beef, veal, and lamb to 145°F (62°C). A meat thermometer can be used to check the temperature of meat. Washing meat does not help. In fact, it can hurt by spreading the bacteria from the meat to other surfaces. In any case, cooking will kill the bacteria. Make sure, also, to wash your hands with antibacterial soap after handling raw meat.

Finally, artificial hormones can be avoided by eating certified organic beef, for example. Milk containing rBGH is labeled in stores, so it is easy to avoid. The USDA-certified organic G label means that the animals were not given any artificial hormones. If meat or dairy is bought from a local farmer, a consumer can just ask if he or she administered any artificial hormones to the animal.

CHANGE IS IN THE WIND

While pesticide use can be problematic, new techniques are being adopted to lower their use. Integrated pest management (IPM) is a method recommended by the EPA, the UN, and ecologists focused on managing and controlling pests. Eradicating entire pest populations is unlikely and impossible. Instead, IPM focuses on establishing acceptable levels of a pest, observing crops, using natural controls—such as insects that are predators for specific pests or beneficial fungi—and, finally, only using pesticides when necessary, as opposed to as a matter of course.

In addition, the FDA is making efforts to phase out the use of medically important antimicrobials—including antibiotics—in animals for the purposes of growth promotion or feed efficiency. Medically important antimicrobials are substances that fight microorganisms in humans with little or no harm to people. This effort aims for drug companies to stop recommending these medications for growth promotion and feed efficiency and to make antimicrobials available only by prescription from a veterinarian. These drugs would then only be given if they were needed to keep an animal healthy and alive, not to make it grow faster. At the moment, this process is voluntary for the companies that make antibiotics, though the FDA says that it is "confident in their support."

The secret to being healthy is not a secret at all. Eat fruits and vegetables that are in season. According to the CDC, only one in ten Americans eats enough of them. Prepare them well, too. Wash all fruits and vegetables, and peel them if necessary. Avoid processed meats and other foods that are full of high-fructose corn syrup. Cook meat thoroughly and understand food safety. Learn where your food comes from, and if you can,

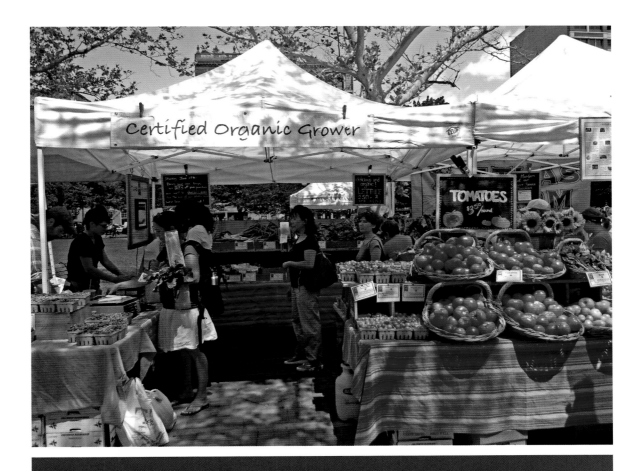

Check and see if there is a farmer's market near you. This way you can be sure you're getting the freshest, healthiest produce from local farms.

ask the producer how it was made. Be informed: avoid making assumptions about what is healthy based on popular knowledge. "Natural," for instance, is a meaningless food label. Meanwhile, "organic" does not necessarily mean that the food is safe. Finally, remember to exercise. Our bodies and brains need it for our physical and mental health.

10 GREAT QUESTIONS
TO ASK A NUTRITIONIST

1. Am I taking antibiotics when I don't really need them?

2. What fruits and vegetables can I replace the EWG's Dirty Dozen with to get the same nutrition?

3. Am I eating enough fruits and vegetables, or should I be eating more?

4. What can I do to minimize exposure to endocrine disruptors?

5. What fish should I eat to avoid the effects of biomagnification?

6. Is a snack that's labeled "all natural" better for me than a non-organic fruit?

7. Should I eat more chicken than beef since chicken is hormone-free?

8. Are the hormones in the dairy products I eat harmful? Should I be eating less dairy?

9. Is eating organic better for my health?

10. Are the quantities of pesticide residue on my fruits and vegetables carcinogenic?

GLOSSARY

antibiotic A substance produced from organisms like bacteria, molds, and fungi to kill or prevent the reproduction of bacteria.

antimicrobial medication A medication used to treat a microbial infection, be it a viral, fungal, or microbial infection. An antibiotic is a kind of antimicrobial.

biochemistry Chemistry of processes and compounds occurring in living organisms.

biomagnification The process whereby a substance increases in concentration the higher it moves up the food chain.

carcinogenic Causing cancer.

cast The nitrogen- and phosphate-containing waste product of earthworms.

contamination The process of making something impure or infected by contact.

endocrine disruptor Chemicals to which our bodies respond like they would to hormones produced by the body itself.

hormone A chemical messenger that regulates various biochemical reactions. In humans, they play an important role in reproduction, growth, and energy regulation.

pesticide Pesticides are substances that prevent, repel, or destroy pests, which can come in the form of insects, weeds, fungi, and rodents.

resistance The natural ability of an organism to survive or avoid a substance that is toxic to it.

synthetic Something produced artificially.

yield The quantity of something, like a crop, produced.

FOR MORE INFORMATION

Canada Food Inspection Agency (CFIA)
1400 Merivale Road
Ottawa, ON K1A 0Y9
Canada
(800) 442-2342
Website: www.inspection.gc.ca
Facebook: @CFIACanada
Twitter: @CFIA_Canada
The CFIA is like the United States' FDA: it is in charge of maintaining and enforcing food standards in Canada that will benefit people, animals, and the environment.

Centers for Disease Control and Prevention (CDC)
1600 Clifton Road
Atlanta, GA 30329
(800) 232-4636
Website: www.cdc.gov
Facebook: @CDC
Twitter: @CDCgov
Instagram: @CDCgov
The CDC gives information on healthy eating, food safety, and what agricultural practices could be potentially threatening to humans.

Environmental Protection Agency (EPA)
1200 Pennsylvania Avenue NW
Washington, DC 20460
(202) 272-0167
Website: www.epa.gov
Facebook: @EPA
Twitter: @EPA
The EPA provides helpful and easy to understand information on

US government policies concerning the effects of pollutants, like pesticides, on our environment.

Food and Drug Administration (FDA)
10903 New Hampshire Avenue
Silver Spring, MD 20993
(888) 463-6332
Website: fda.gov
Facebook: @FDA
Twitter: @US_FDA
YouTube: USFoodandDrugAdmin
The FDA is in charge of regulating the foods we eat and how they are produced. Their website provides information on current government policies concerning agricultural practices.

Health Canada
Address Locator 0900C2
Ottawa, ON K1A 0K9
Canada
(613) 957-2991
Website: http://www.hc-sc.gc.ca
Facebook: @HealthyCdns
Twitter: @HealthCanada
Health Canada is a federal department that works with the CFIA to provide information about food and animals, current practices and policies, and potential health hazards, as well as advice for healthy living.

National Resource Defense Council (NRDC)
40 West 20th Street, 11th Floor
New York, NY 10011
(212) 727-2700
Website: www.nrdc.org

Facebook: @NRDC.org
Twitter: @NRDC
Instagram: @NRDC_org
The NRDC is an organization devoted to protecting our environment. They have multiple focuses, among them food and agricultural practices that could be harmful, as well as suggestions for staying healthy and aware.

WEBSITES

Because of the changing nature of internet links, Rosen Publishing has developed an online list of websites related to the subject of this book. This site is updated regularly. Please use this link to access the list:

http://www.rosenlinks.com/FFTT/Pest

FOR FURTHER READING

Barker, David. *Organic Foods*. Minneapolis, MN: Lerner Publications, 2016.

Carson, Rachel. *Silent Spring*. Boston, MA: Houghton Mifflin Harcourt, 2002.

Hughes, Meredith Sayles. *Plants vs. Meats: The Health, History, and Ethics of What We Eat*. Minneapolis, MN: Twenty-First Century Books, 2016.

Hurt, Avery Elizabeth, ed. *Corporate Farming* (Opposing Viewpoints). New York, NY: Greenhaven Publishing, 2018.

Miller, Debra A., ed. *Pesticides* (Current Controversies). Farmington Hills, MI: Greenhaven Press, 2014.

Pollan, Michael. *Food Rules*. New York, NY: Penguin Press, 2011.

Quinlan, Julia J., and Watson, Stephanie. *The Truth Behind Manufactured Meats*. New York, NY: Rosen Central, 2018.

Regis, Natalie, ed. *Genetically Modified Crops and Food* (The Biotechnology Revolution). New York, NY: Britannica Educational Publishing, 2016.

Rissman, Rebecca, and Susan Oh. *Eating Organic* (Food Matters). Minneapolis, MN: ABDO Publishing, 2016.

BIBLIOGRAPHY

Alavanja, Michael C. R., Jane A. Hoppin, and Freya Kamel. "Health Effects of Chronic Pesticide Exposure: Cancer and Neurotoxicity." *Annual Review of Public Health* (25) (2004): 155-197. Retrieved March 20, 2017. doi: 10.1146/annurev. publhealth.25.101802.123020.

Centers for Disease Control. "About DES." Retrieved March 15, 2017. https://www.cdc.gov/des/consumers/about/history.html.

Edwards, Clive A. "Earthworms." Natural Resources Conservation Service. Retrieved April 2, 2017. https://www.nrcs.usda .gov/wps/portal/nrcs/detailfull/soils/health/biology/?cid =nrcs142p2_053863.

Environmental Protection Agency. "Introduction to Integrated Pest Management." Retrieved April 3, 2017. https://www .epa.gov/managing-pests-schools/introduction-integrated -pest-management.

European Commission. "Pesticides and Bees." Retrieved April 1, 2017. https://ec.europa.eu/food/animals/live_animals/bees /pesticides_en.

Food and Drug Administration. "FDA's Strategy on Antimicrobial Resistance: Questions and Answers." February 14, 2017. https://www.fda.gov/animalveterinary /guidancecomplianceenforcement/guidanceforindustry /ucm216939.htm.

Foodsafety.gov. "Charts: Food Safety at a Glance." Retrieved April 3, 2017. https://www.foodsafety.gov/keep/charts /mintemp.html.

Jolly, David. "Europe Bans Pesticides Thought Harmful to Bees." *New York Times*, April 29, 2013. http://www.nytimes .com/2013/04/30/business/global/30iht-eubees30.html.

Maron, Dina Fine. "Early Puberty: Causes and Effects." *Scientific American*, May 1, 2015.

Pearson, Gwen. "Pesticides and Bees: It's Complex." *Wired*,

March 18, 2015. https://www.wired.com/2015/03/pesticides
-bees-complex.

Royal Holloway, University of London. "Exposure to pesticides
results in smaller worker bees." ScienceDaily. Retrieved April
2, 2017. https://www.sciencedaily.com/releases/2014/01
/140120090643.htm.

Takamiya Allen, Minako, and Leonard S. Levy. "Parkinson's Disease and Pesticide Exposure: A New Assessment." *Critical
Reviews in Toxicology* (43) (2013): 515–34. Retrieved March
20, 2017. doi: 10.3109/10408444.2013.798719. February 19,
2017. https://www.scientificamerican.com/article/early
-puberty-causes-and-effects/.

University of Southern Denmark. "Pesticides make the life of
earthworms miserable." ScienceDaily, March 25, 2014. https://
www.sciencedaily.com/releases/2014/03/140325113232.htm.

Weil, Elizabeth. "Puberty Before Age 10: A New Normal?" *New
York Times Magazine*, March 30, 2012. http://www.nytimes
.com/2012/04/01/magazine/puberty-before-age-10-a-new
-normal.html.

Wilcox, Christie. "Are Lower Pesticide Residues a Good Reason
to Buy Organic? Probably Not." *Scientific American*, September 24, 2012. https://blogs.scientificamerican.com/science
-sushi/pesticides-food-fears.

INDEX

A

antibiotic-resistant bacteria, 10, 16, 18, 20, 23
antibiotics
  discovery of, 8
  effects on animals, 10
  effects of humans, 16, 18
  medicine, 7–9
  resistance to, 10, 16, 18, 20, 23
antimicrobials, 36

B

bacteria, 10, 16–17, 18–20, 35
bacterial infections, 9, 10, 18–20
bees, 26–29
bioaccumulation, 24, 26
biomagnification, 25
bisphenol A (BPA), 23

C

Campylobacter, 18, 19
Campylobacteriosis, 19
cancer, 11, 21, 22, 23, 31
Carson, Rachel, 25
Centers for Disease Control and Prevention (CDC), 10, 21, 35, 36
copper sulfate, 33–34

D

diabetes, type 2, 11
dichloro-diphenyl-trychloroethane (DDT), 25–26, 33
diethylstilbestrol (DES), 21

E

earthworms, 26, 29–30
endocrine disruptors (EDs), 11, 14, 20–23, 31
endocrine system, 20, 23, 26
Environmental Protection Agency (EPA), 11, 20, 26, 36
Environmental Working Group (EWG), 32, 33
Escherichia coli (E. coli), 18
estrogen, 15, 21, 22, 23
European Union (EU), 13, 27

F

Fleming, Alexander, 8
Florey, Howard, 9
Food and Drug Administration (FDA), 21, 26, 36

G

growth-promoting antibiotics (GPAs), 10

H

hormones
  effects on animals, 12
  effects on the environment, 26
  risk to humans, 20–21
  synthetic, 14

I

insecticide, 10, 25, 27, 28, 29
integrated pest management (IPM), 36

ABOUT THE AUTHOR

Katharina Smundak is a writer and English teacher living in France.

PHOTO CREDITS